THE CANCER WAR

A Comprehensive Guide to Understanding, Managing, and Enhancing Physical Wellness.

By

Brian A. Godfrey

TABLE OF CONTENTS

INTRODUCTION

Millions of people worldwide are impacted by the complicated and dangerous disease known as cancer, which poses a constant challenge to the medical profession. We shall explore the complexities of cancer in this article, including its description, underlying causes, risk factors, and the many forms that affect various body regions. We can develop efficient methods for cancer prevention, diagnosis, and therapy by developing a thorough understanding of the disease.

Cancer: What Is It?

Cancer is a collective term for a class of disorders defined by aberrant cells within the body growing and dividing out of control. In contrast to healthy cells, which divide and multiply randomly and carry out particular tasks, cancer cells divide and proliferate uncontrollably, giving rise to malignant tumors or, through a process called metastasis, spreading to other areas of the body. Unchecked growth has the potential to disrupt the regular operations of tissues and organs, resulting in various health concerns.

Causes and Risk Factors

A number of variables have a role in the development of cancer, even though its precise causes are numerous and frequently complex. These variables may be roughly divided into two groups: those that are changeable and those that are not.

Modifiable risk factors:
a. Lifestyle decisions: A person's risk of developing cancer can be considerably increased by making certain lifestyle decisions, such as using tobacco products, drinking too much alcohol, eating an unhealthy diet low in fruits and vegetables,

being sedentary, and being exposed to dangerous chemicals or substances.

b. Sun Exposure: Extended sun exposure or the use of artificial tanning beds can raise your chance of developing skin cancer.

c. Infections: A higher risk of developing some cancers has been associated with bacterial and viral infections, including Helicobacter pylori (H. pylori) infection, hepatitis B and C, and human papillomavirus (HPV).

2. Non-changeable risk elements:
a. Genetic Predisposition: Gene mutations passed down via inheritance may raise the risk of getting some cancers. It is crucial to remember that other environmental and lifestyle variables also play a big part in cancer development; therefore, genetic predisposition does not ensure that cancer will occur.

b. Age: As we age, our bodies' natural defenses and healing processes may become less effective, which raises our chance of acquiring cancer.

c. Family History: An individual's risk for several forms of cancer may be somewhat increased if they have a close relative, such as a parent or sibling, who has a history of the disease.

Types of Cancer

The disease can affect any organ, tissue, or system in the body, and it can take many distinct forms. These are a few prevalent cancer types:

1. Carcinomas: The most common kind of cancer, carcinomas are caused by the epithelial cells that encircle the organs and tissues of the body. Prostate, colon, lung, and breast cancers are a few examples.

2. Sarcomas: Sarcomas arise in the soft tissues, muscles, and connective tissues. Osteosarcoma and leiomyosarcoma are two examples.

3. Leukemias: These malignancies of the bone marrow and blood cause an excessive production of white blood cells. Acute lymphoblastic leukemia (ALL) and chronic myeloid leukemia (CML) are two examples.

4. Lymphomas: The lymphatic system, which is made up of the spleen, bone marrow, and lymph nodes, is where lymphomas develop. Non-Hodgkin lymphoma and Hodgkin lymphoma are two examples.

5. Central Nervous System (CNS) Tumors: These tumors can be malignant or benign and arise in the brain or spinal cord. Gliomas and medulloblastomas are two examples. In summary, cancer is a multifaceted illness that results from

aberrant cells in the body growing out of
control. We may lower our risk, encourage
early identification, and pursue the
necessary medical procedures by being
aware of the nature of cancer and its
causes, risk factors, and different forms.
The continued battle against cancer
depends heavily on research, treatment
techniques, and preventative education. As
a society, we can work toward better results,
higher standards of living, and eventually a
future free from the terrifying menace of
cancer.

Part I: Prevention and Risk Reduction

Lifestyle Factors and Cancer Prevention

The Role of Diet and Nutrition

The prevention of cancer is greatly influenced by diet and nutrition, as ongoing research reveals the deep influence that food choices have on our general health and wellbeing. A balanced diet high in nutrient-dense foods and low in processed and unhealthy foods can dramatically lower the chance of developing cancer, even if genetics and environmental factors still play a role. The main ideas of a cancer-preventive diet will be discussed in this section, along with particular foods and dietary habits that have been demonstrated to reduce the chance of developing certain cancers.

1. Place a Focus on Plant-Based Foods:
Including a wide range of plant-based foods in one's diet is essential for preventing cancer. These include fruits, vegetables, whole grains, legumes, nuts, and seeds. It has been demonstrated that the abundance of vitamins, minerals, antioxidants, and phytochemicals in these meals has anti-cancer effects. Eat as many different colors of fruits and vegetables as you can, including berries, leafy greens, carrots, bell peppers, and cruciferous vegetables like Brussels sprouts, broccoli, and cauliflower.

2. Cut Back on Processed and Red Meats:
Prostate, pancreatic, and colorectal cancers have all been associated with a high red and processed meat intake. Saturated lipids and heme iron are found in red meats like lamb, hog, and cattle, which may hasten the onset of cancer. Bacon, sausage, hot dogs,

and deli meats are examples of processed meats that frequently include preservatives and chemicals that have been linked to cancer. Limit your consumption of these meats and choose leaner protein sources like beans, lentils, fish, chicken, and tofu to lower your risk of cancer.

3. Pick Good Fats:
Include healthy fats in your diet, such as those in nuts, seeds, avocados, olive oil, and fatty fish like sardines and salmon. These fats include monounsaturated and omega-3 fatty acids, which have anti-inflammatory qualities and may help lower the risk of several malignancies. Trans and saturated fats, which are included in processed and fried foods, should be avoided or consumed in moderation since they have been linked to an increased risk of heart disease and several types of cancer.

4. Boost Your Fiber Consumption:

Whole grains, fruits, vegetables, legumes, and other foods high in fiber are essential for preserving digestive health and lowering the risk of colorectal cancer. Constipation is avoided, regular bowel movements are encouraged, and the digestive system is kept healthy with the aid of fiber. Aim to eat a range of foods high in fiber, such as cruciferous vegetables, apples, pears, quinoa, brown rice, beans, lentils, and oats.

5. Keep Your Water Up:

In addition to being vital for general health, enough hydration may help prevent cancer. Water supports cellular processes, helps remove toxins from the body, and helps control body temperature. Try to stay hydrated during the day by drinking lots of water and consuming as few sugar-filled liquids as possible, such as fruit juice, soda, and energy drinks.

6. Consider Portions Carefully

To prevent overeating and preserve a healthy weight, choose foods high in nutrients and be mindful of portion sizes. The chance of developing breast, colorectal, pancreatic, and kidney cancers has been associated with obesity and excess body fat. Eat with awareness, enjoying every meal, and stopping when you're full rather than full.

7. Look for Expert Advice:

The nutritional requirements of an individual may differ depending on age, gender, degree of exercise, and pre-existing medical issues. Consider speaking with a licensed dietitian or nutritionist if you have special dietary problems or are unaware of how to best prepare your food for cancer prevention. They can offer individualized advice and suggestions that are tailored to your requirements and tastes.

Importance of Physical Activity

Engaging in physical activity is an essential part of maintaining a healthy lifestyle and is particularly important in preventing cancer. Frequent exercise directly affects several biological processes in the body that can lower the chance of developing cancer, in addition to aiding in the maintenance of a healthy weight. This section will discuss the role that physical activity plays in preventing cancer and offer helpful advice on how to fit exercise into your daily schedule.

1. Sustaining an Appropriate Weight:

A healthy weight is crucial for cancer prevention and must be attained and maintained via regular physical exercise. Excess body fat and obesity have been associated with a higher risk of colon, pancreatic, renal, and breast cancers, among other malignancies. In addition to lowering cancer risk and helping people maintain their weight, exercise also helps people burn calories, gain lean muscle mass, and enhance metabolic health.

2. Diminishing Inflammation:

It is thought that chronic inflammation contributes to the formation of tumors, DNA damage, and cell proliferation in cancer. Frequent exercise helps lower levels of inflammatory markers and cytokines linked to an increased risk of cancer by having anti-inflammatory effects on the body. Physical exercise may help prevent cancer from starting and spreading by reducing systemic inflammation.

3. Enhancing the Immune System:

The immune system is essential for locating and destroying malignant cells before they have a chance to develop into tumors. It has been demonstrated that physical exercise improves immune function by raising the generation and activation of immune cells such macrophages, T cells, and natural killer cells. Frequent exercise may enhance immune surveillance and the body's reaction to cancer cells, hence lowering the risk of cancer initiation and progression.

4. Maintaining Hormone Balance:

The development of cancer is significantly influenced by hormones, especially hormone-sensitive malignancies like prostate and breast cancer. Insulin, estrogen, and testosterone levels in the body may all be regulated by physical exercise, potentially lowering the incidence of hormone-related malignancies. Exercise has been shown to decrease circulating estrogen levels, increase insulin sensitivity, and modify sex hormone-binding globulin (SHBG), all of which are protective against cancer.

6. Improving Mental Health:

Engaging in physical activity has advantages for both mental and physical health. Exercise on a regular basis has been demonstrated to lower stress, anxiety, and depression—all of which are linked to a higher risk of cancer and other chronic illnesses. Exercise has been shown to enhance overall quality of life and indirectly lessen the risk of cancer by improving mental health and lowering psychological discomfort.

7. Useful Advice for Increasing Exercise: It's not necessary to make incorporating exercise into your everyday routine difficult or time-consuming. Set attainable goals in the beginning and work your way up to longer and more intense workouts. Aim for 75 minutes of strenuous activity or at least 150 minutes of moderate-intensity aerobic activity each week, in addition to two or more days of muscle-strengthening activities.

Here are some doable suggestions to boost physical activity:
- Going for vigorous walks during your lunch break or just after dinner; - Choosing to walk or cycle small distances rather than drive
- Engaging in leisure sports or group fitness courses; - Whenever feasible, choose the stairs over elevators; - Including strength training activities with resistance bands or body weight.

Avoiding Harmful Substances

One of the most important aspects of cancer prevention is limiting exposure to dangerous chemicals. Carcinogens, environmental pollutants, and other dangerous elements present in commonplace goods and activities can raise the chance of developing cancer. Through proactive measures to minimize exposure and awareness of possible dangers, people can lower their risk of cancer and improve their general health and well-being. This section will discuss common dangerous compounds to stay away from and offer helpful advice on how to reduce exposure in day-to-day activities.

1. Smoke from tobacco:

Thousands of compounds, many of which are recognized carcinogens that can harm DNA and raise the risk of cancer, are found in tobacco smoke. Smoking is closely associated with lung, throat, oral, esophageal, bladder, and pancreatic cancers and is the primary avoidable cause of cancer-related deaths globally. One of the best methods to lower the risk of cancer is to avoid being around tobacco smoke, either by smoking yourself or by watching others smoke.

2. Intake of Alcohol:

Drinking too much alcohol is linked to a higher chance of developing breast, liver, colorectal, esophageal, and oral cancers, among other malignancies. Through a number of pathways, such as a weakened immune system, inflammation, and damage to DNA, alcohol can encourage the development of cancer. Reducing alcohol use to moderate levels (one drink for women and two for men) or giving it up completely can help lower the risk of cancer and enhance general health outcomes.

3. Radiation from Ultraviolet Sources: UV radiation exposure from the sun and artificial sources, including tanning beds, can damage skin and raise the chance of developing skin cancer, which includes squamous cell carcinoma, basal cell carcinoma, and melanoma. Skin cancer can be prevented and skin health can be enhanced by shielding your skin from UV radiation using sunscreen, protective clothes, and sunglasses, finding shade during the hottest parts of the day, and refraining from indoor tanning.

4. Carcinogens in the Environment:
The chance of developing cancer can be raised by exposure to environmental carcinogens, including industrial chemicals, asbestos, arsenic, benzene, and air pollution. These compounds can be found in polluted water supplies, home items, outdoor air pollution, and work environments. Cancer risk can be decreased and public health can be safeguarded by minimizing exposure to environmental carcinogens through appropriate ventilation, protective gear, and adherence to safety laws.

5. Chemicals and Pesticides in Food:
Chemicals and pesticides left behind after food production can be harmful to human health and eventually raise the chance of developing cancer. One way to reduce your exposure to dangerous compounds in food is to choose organic produce wherever feasible, wash fruits and vegetables well

before eating them, and stay away from processed meals that include artificial additives and preservatives.

6. Disruptors of Hormone and Endocrine Systems:

Hormonal and endocrine disruptors, a class of chemicals included in consumer goods, plastics, and personal hygiene products, can alter hormone function and raise the risk of hormone-related malignancies, including breast and prostate cancer. Reducing exposure to these hazardous compounds can be achieved by avoiding goods that include phthalates, parabens, bisphenol A (BPA), and other known endocrine disruptors; instead, choosing natural and chemical-free alternatives; and storing food and beverages in glass or stainless steel containers.

7. Gas Radon:

Radon is a naturally occurring radioactive gas that can cause lung cancer because it can enter buildings through foundational fissures and build up within. By having your house tested for radon and putting mitigation measures in place, such as installing radon mitigation systems, sealing gaps, and optimizing airflow, you may help lower exposure and prevent lung cancer.

Screening and Early Detection

Importance of Regular Screening

Reducing mortality, increasing overall survival, and improving treatment results all depend on the early diagnosis of cancer through routine screening. Screening tests can find cancer early on, typically before symptoms appear, when it is most curable. Early cancer detection allows medical professionals to respond quickly with the right treatment plans, perhaps stopping the disease's development and improving patient outcomes. This section will discuss the significance of routinely screening for different cancer types and highlight important screening criteria and recommendations.

1. Early Cancer Identification:

Frequent screening exams are intended to find precancerous alterations or cancer in people who do not exhibit illness signs. Prompt diagnosis and treatment are made possible by early detection, which can greatly increase the likelihood of positive results. Early-stage discovery by screening can improve the prognosis and lessen the need for harsh therapies for a number of cancers, including colorectal, prostate, cervical, and breast cancer.

2. Enhancing Therapy Results:

Healthcare professionals can use prompt and suitable therapeutic approaches, including surgery, chemotherapy, radiation therapy, and targeted therapies, when cancer is detected early. Compared to advanced-stage illnesses, early-stage cancer therapy options are frequently less intrusive and have fewer adverse effects. Early intervention may also stop cancer from spreading to other body areas, which would enhance the effectiveness of treatment and prolong survival.

3. Lowering Death Rates:

Frequent screening has been demonstrated to lower the death rates of several cancer types by finding cancers when they are still more curable. For instance, screening mammography has been linked to a noteworthy reduction in the death rate from breast cancer, and screening colonoscopy can save lives from colorectal cancer by identifying and eliminating precancerous polyps. Screening programs have the potential to prevent cancer-related fatalities and save lives by detecting the disease early and starting the right therapy.

4. Recognizing People at High Risk:

Additionally, screening tests can assist in identifying those who are more susceptible to cancer because of hereditary or family causes. To identify those at high risk of hereditary breast and ovarian cancer, for instance, genetic testing for BRCA1 and BRCA2 mutations can be used. This enables focused surveillance and preventative action. Screening recommendations have the potential to facilitate early diagnosis and intervention in high-risk groups by recommending earlier or more frequent screenings for people with established risk factors.

5. Using Knowledge to Empower Patients:

By educating people about their cancer risk and early warning indicators, routine screenings enable people to actively participate in their health and wellbeing. People can proactively monitor their health status and collaborate with healthcare practitioners to address any concerns or anomalies discovered during screening tests by taking part in screening programs and following prescribed procedures. Patients who receive early detection through screening are able to explore suitable treatment choices based on their own needs and preferences and make educated decisions regarding their care.

6. Adhering to Suggested Screening Protocols

People must adhere to screening recommendations depending on their age, gender, family history, and other risk factors. Depending on the type of cancer and a person's unique risk profile, different screening guidelines may apply. Healthcare professionals may offer advice on the advantages and restrictions of screening tests as well as assist in determining the best screening plan for each patient. People can lessen their chance of acquiring advanced-stage cancer and optimize the possible advantages of early diagnosis by following advice and being screened on a regular basis.

Common Screening Tests

Screening tests are effective instruments in the battle against cancer because they allow abnormalities or malignant alterations to be found early, before symptoms appear. Early cancer detection allows medical professionals to start treatments on time, which improves treatment results and increases survival rates. This section will examine some frequently used screening tests for cancer early detection and address their significance in cancer prevention initiatives.

1. Screening for breast cancer using mammography:
Mammography is a commonly used breast cancer screening test that is usually advised

for women 40 years of age and older. Low-dose X-rays are utilized during a mammogram to find anomalies in the breast tissue, such as cancers or microcalcifications. Frequent mammograms have the potential to lower death rates and increase long-term survival by detecting breast cancer at an early stage, when it is most curable.

2. Cervical Cancer Screening with Pap Smear:

A Pap smear, often referred to as a Pap test, is a cervical cancer screening procedure that entails removing cells from the cervix and looking for anomalies under a microscope. Early intervention and therapy are made possible by the Pap smear's ability to identify precancerous alterations in cervical cells brought on by human papillomavirus (HPV) infection. Pap smears are a highly effective way to lower the incidence of cervical cancer and reduce deaths attributable to cancer when combined with HPV testing.

3. Colonoscopy: A Screening for Colorectal Cancer:

Colonoscopy, which uses a long, flexible tube with a camera to look for abnormal growths called polyps inside the colon and rectum, is the gold standard for screening for colorectal cancer. Any polyps found during the treatment might be extracted and biopsied to find out if they are precancerous or cancerous. Colonoscopy is a highly successful screening tool for lowering colorectal cancer death rates since it may identify the disease early or completely prevent it by eliminating precancerous polyps.

4. Prostate-Specific Antigen (PSA) Test for Screening for Prostate Cancer:

Prostate-specific antigen, a protein generated by the prostate gland, is measured in the blood via the PSA test.

Prostate cancer and other diseases connected to the prostate may be detected by elevated PSA levels, which would require further testing, such as a digital rectal exam or prostate biopsy. The PSA test is still a useful tool for the early identification of prostate cancer in some groups, especially men who are at high risk or have symptoms that may indicate prostate cancer, despite its contentious nature stemming from worries about overdiagnosis and overtreatment.

5. Screening for Skin Cancer:

A medical professional will thoroughly examine your skin during a skin cancer screening in order to look for any abnormal lesions, moles, or changes in the texture or color of your skin that might point to the disease. Frequent skin self-examinations and professional skin examinations can aid in the early detection of both melanoma and non-melanoma skin cancers, when treatment options are most favorable. Skin cancer screening is a vital part of preventative healthcare since early diagnosis of skin cancer is necessary for successful treatment and better results.

6. Screening for Lung Cancer:

People who have a high risk of acquiring lung cancer, usually those who have smoked heavily in the past and are between the ages of 50 and 80, should get screened for the disease. Low-dose computed tomography (CT) scanning is the most popular screening test for lung cancer because it can find anomalies or lung nodules that could be signs of early-stage lung cancer. Particularly for those who are at a high risk of the illness, early identification of lung cancer by screening may result in earlier treatment and higher survival rates.

Early Warning Signs of Cancer

Early cancer detection is essential for a timely diagnosis and course of treatment. Although screening tests are necessary to identify cancer in its early stages, people may speed up early diagnosis and seek medical assistance by being aware of common symptoms and indicators. This section will address some of the early indicators of cancer that people should be aware of, as well as the significance of being checked out by a doctor if you have any worrisome symptoms.

1. Inexplicable Loss of Weight:

Unexpected weight loss, especially if it's substantial and accidental and weighs 10 pounds or more, may indicate a number of diseases, including stomach, lung, esophageal, and pancreatic cancers. Cancer-related weight loss can be brought on by a variety of conditions, including decreased appetite, altered metabolism, or the existence of tumors that drain the body's nutrition and energy.

2. Extended Exhaustion:

Excessive or chronic fatigue that does not go away with rest may be an indication of cancer or some other underlying medical issue. Fatigue associated with cancer may be caused by anemia, inflammation, or the immune system's reaction to cancerous cells. Cancer-related fatigue can be crippling and interfere with day-to-day activities, which can lower quality of life and negatively impact general wellbeing.

3. Modifications to Bladder or Bowel Habits:

Prostate, colorectal, or bladder cancer may be indicated by changes in bowel or bladder habits, such as recurrent diarrhea, constipation, blood in the urine or stool, or changes in the frequency or urgency of urinating. These symptoms might indicate the need for additional testing by a medical professional since they could be caused by tumors or other anomalies in the gastrointestinal or urinary tract.

4. Chronic Illness:

Unbearable or chronic pain that does not go away with time or medication may be an early indicator of cancer. The location and degree of cancer-related pain might vary based on the disease's kind and stage. Bone pain (from bone metastases), pelvic or abdominal pain (from malignancies of the reproductive organs), and headaches or neurological pain (from brain tumors) are common locations of cancer-related pain.

5. Skin Changes:

A dermatologist should be seen for any changes to the skin, including moles that have grown or changed, non-healing wounds, and modifications to the size, shape, or color of preexisting lesions. These alterations might be a sign of skin cancer, especially melanoma, which is the most fatal kind. In order to stop the illness from spreading and to improve the prognosis, early identification and treatment of skin cancer are essential.

6. Prolonged Cough or Hoarse Voice:
Hoarseness, voice quality changes, or a chronic cough that lasts longer than a few weeks might indicate an underlying throat or respiratory malignancy. Other respiratory symptoms, including wheezing, chest discomfort, or shortness of breath, may accompany these symptoms. People who have ongoing respiratory problems should contact a doctor to rule out other possible illnesses, such as cancer.

7. Density or Swelling:
A healthcare professional should be consulted right away if there is a lump or thickening in the breast, testicle, lymph nodes, or any other portion of the body. Even though not every bump is malignant, more research to identify its etiology may be

necessary. Testicular lumps may be an indication of testicular cancer, whereas breast lumps may be suggestive of breast cancer. Expanded lymph nodes might also be a sign that cancer has migrated from a main tumor to another part of the body.

Part II: Treatment Options

Traditional Treatments

Surgery: Types and Procedures

One of the main therapeutic approaches used to treat different kinds of cancer is surgery. To stop or slow the spread of cancer, it entails removing malignant tissue and, occasionally, adjacent lymph nodes or organs. Highly sophisticated surgical techniques are used to treat cancer, and the specifics of each patient, the kind and stage of the disease, and the location of the tumor can all affect the outcome. This section will discuss common procedures, surgical approaches used to treat cancer, and things to think about before having surgery.

Surgical Types:
1. Surgical Correction: In order to cure the cancer or achieve a long-term remission,

the goal of curative surgery is to remove the
whole tumor along with any surrounding
tissue. It is frequently applied to early-stage
malignancies that have not migrated to
other body areas and are localized.

2. Surgical Debulking: When eliminating
the full tumor is not feasible, debulking
surgery entails removing a section of the
tumor. This technique can be carried out to
reduce symptoms, enhance quality of life, or
increase the efficacy of other therapies,
such as radiation therapy or chemotherapy.
3. Surgical Palliative Care: Patients with
advanced-stage cancer can benefit from
palliative surgery by having their symptoms
lessened or their quality of life enhanced. To
relieve pain or suffering, it can entail
removing tumors, releasing obstructions, or
compressing surrounding tissues, such as
blood vessels or nerves.

Typical Surgical Techniques:

1. Breast Cancer Surgery: Lumpectomy or Mastectomy: A mastectomy entails removing the entire breast during treatment for breast cancer, whereas a lumpectomy just removes the tumor and a small margin of surrounding tissue. Tumor size, location, and patient preference are among the criteria that influence the surgical method decision.

2. Hysterectomy (Cancer Surgery of the Uterus or Ovaries): For the treatment of ovarian or uterine cancer, a hysterectomy may be performed to remove the uterus (total hysterectomy) or the uterus and cervix (total hysterectomy with bilateral salpingo-oophorectomy). In certain instances, excision of the ovaries and fallopian tubes may also be necessary to lower the chance of cancer returning.

3. Surgery for prostate cancer: Prostatectomy In order to treat prostate cancer, a prostatectomy entails the surgical removal of the prostate gland. The technique may be carried out by open surgery, laparoscopic surgery, or robotic-assisted laparoscopic surgery, depending on the severity of the condition.

4. Colectomy (Surgery for Colorectal Cancer): A colonectomy is the surgical excision of a colorectal cancer-affected part of the colon or rectum. A stoma (colostomy or ileostomy) may be created to remove waste from the body, or the tumor and surrounding lymph nodes may be removed, and the healthy sections of the colon or rectum may be rejoined (anastomosis).

5. Lymph Node Dissection: In order to determine whether cancer has progressed to the lymphatic system, lymph nodes in the vicinity of the main tumor are surgically removed. In order to ascertain the degree of disease dissemination and inform subsequent treatment options, it is frequently carried out in tandem with other cancer procedures.

Thoughts for Patients Having Surgery: 1. Initial Assessment: Patients will go through a thorough preoperative assessment before surgery in order to evaluate their general health, find any coexisting diseases, and establish their surgical suitability. Consultations with specialists, imaging examinations, and laboratory testing may be necessary for this.

2. Dangers and Consequences of Surgery: Complications with cancer surgery include bleeding, infection, anesthetic responses, and injury to adjacent tissues, just like with any surgical treatment. Before surgery, patients should address any worries or inquiries with their healthcare staff and go over the possible risks and advantages.

3. Rehabilitation and Recovery: Patients will need time for recuperation and rehabilitation after surgery in order to restore function and strength. This might entail dietary changes, physical therapy, wound care, and pain management. Patients should adhere to the postoperative recommendations given by their medical team and show up for follow-up appointments on time.

4. Supplemental Treatment: Adjuvant therapy, such as chemotherapy, radiation therapy, or targeted therapy, may be used in some situations after surgery to treat residual illness or lower the chance of cancer recurrence. Depending on variables including the features of the tumor, the disease's stage, and the results of the surgery, adjuvant therapy may be suggested.

Chemotherapy: How It Works and Side Effects

One common cancer treatment method is chemotherapy, which tries to either kill cancer cells or stop them from growing and spreading throughout the body. It entails the use of potent pharmaceuticals called "cytotoxic drugs," which target cells that divide quickly, particularly cancer cells. Chemotherapy can be useful in eliminating cancer cells, but it can also harm healthy cells in the body and cause a number of unfavorable side effects. This section will cover typical side effects, how chemotherapy works, kinds of chemotherapy medications, and techniques to manage adverse effects.

The Mechanism of Chemotherapy:
Chemotherapy targets fast-dividing cells, which are a feature common to cancerous cells. Chemotherapy medications can damage DNA, prevent protein synthesis, or

interfere with other vital cellular processes by interfering with the process of cell division, which eventually results in cell death. Various methods of administering chemotherapy are available, such as oral (by tablets or capsules) or intravenously (via injections or infusions), contingent upon the particular medications and treatment plan.

Drugs Used in Chemotherapy:
1. Alkylating Substances: By introducing alkyl groups to DNA, these medications stop cancer cells from proliferating and dividing. Temozolomide, cisplatin, and cyclophosphamide are a few examples.

2. Antimetabolites: Antimetabolites imitate the structure of nucleotides to interfere with DNA and RNA production, stopping cancer cells from proliferating. Methotrexate, 5-fluorouracil (5-FU), and gemcitabine are a few examples.

3. Antibiotics against Tumors: These medications cause cell death by preventing DNA synthesis or damaging DNA. Doxorubicin, bleomycin, and mitomycin are a few examples.

4. Plant Alkaloids: Plant alkaloids target microtubules, which are structures necessary for cell replication, in order to impair cell division. Paclitaxel, vincristine, and vinblastine are a few examples.

5. Inhibitors of Topoisomerase: Topoisomerase inhibitors prevent the action of topoisomerases, an enzyme that aids in unwinding DNA during cell division. Irinotecan and etoposide are two examples.

Common Chemotherapy Side Effects:
1. Vomiting and Nausea: Chemotherapy medications have the potential to irritate the intestinal and stomach linings, which can cause nausea and vomiting. Antiemetics, or

anti-nausea drugs, may be recommended to treat these symptoms.

2. Exhaustion: Chemotherapy patients may experience significant weariness or exhaustion that lasts for the course of treatment and recovery. Rest, energy conservation, and a little physical exercise are advised for patients as tolerated.

3. Alopecia (loss of hair): Numerous chemotherapy medications have the potential to induce hair loss or thinning, including body, lash, eyebrow, and scalp hair. Often, hair loss is transient and can be reversed when therapy is finished.

4. Suppression of Bone Marrow: Chemotherapy has the ability to reduce bone marrow function, which can result in anemia (low blood cell production), neutropenia (increased risk of infection), and thrombocytopenia (increased risk of bleeding). Regular blood tests can be conducted to track blood cell counts, and supportive care interventions can be put in place as needed.

5. Mucositis (mouth sores):

Chemotherapy medications can cause harm to the gastrointestinal system, throat, and mouth lining, which can result in painful ulcers or mouth sores. Mucositis can be prevented or managed by the use of oral hygiene practices such as gentle brushing and rinsing with saline solution.

6. Decrease in Hunger: Chemotherapy may have an impact on taste and appetite, which might result in less food being consumed and weight loss. Maintaining appropriate nutrition throughout treatment can be facilitated by eating small, frequent meals, drinking enough water, and ingesting nutrient-dense foods.

7. Neuropathy in the Periphery: Certain chemotherapy medications have the potential to harm nerves, which can result in peripheral neuropathy, which manifests as tingling, numbness, or weakness in the hands and feet. After therapy is finished, symptoms could get better, although neuropathy can often linger or get worse over time.

Controlling Adverse Effects:
1. Supportive Care: During chemotherapy treatment, supportive care treatments, including blood transfusions, pain management, and anti-nausea drugs, may be recommended to reduce side effects and enhance quality of life.

2. Dietary Assistance: In addition to food recommendations and nutritional supplements, registered dietitians may offer advice on how to manage taste alterations and appetite loss while undergoing chemotherapy.

3. Physical Activity: During chemotherapy treatment, frequent physical activity can help preserve physical function, lessen tiredness, and enhance mood. Examples of this activity include walking, stretching, and mild workouts.

4. Social Assistance: Patients may benefit from counseling, support groups, or other psychosocial therapies to manage anxiety, depression, or other emotional difficulties, as cancer treatment can be emotionally taxing.

Radiation Therapy: Techniques and Considerations

One popular cancer treatment option is radiation therapy, commonly referred to as radiotherapy. High-energy radiation beams are used in this procedure to target and eliminate cancer cells with the least amount of harm to the surrounding healthy tissues. To get the best possible results, radiation therapy can be performed either alone or in conjunction with other therapies like chemotherapy and surgery. In this part, we will look at the methods and factors related to radiation therapy for the treatment of cancer.

Radiation Therapy Techniques:
1. External Beam Radiation Therapy (EBRT): High-energy radiation beams are delivered directly to the tumor and surrounding tissues via an external beam radiation treatment system. It is the most popular kind of radiation therapy used to treat cancer and can be administered in a number of ways, such as:

3D Conformal Radiation Therapy (3D-CRT): 3D-CRT accurately targets the tumor while avoiding radiation exposure to surrounding healthy tissues. It does this by using sophisticated imaging techniques like computed tomography (CT) or magnetic resonance imaging (MRI).

Radiation Therapy with Intensity Modulated Release (IMRT): With the use of intensely concentrated radiation beams that may be directed and intensified to precisely fit the contours of the tumor, IMRT provides accurate dosing while sparing adjacent vital structures.

Radiotherapy guided by images (IGRT): To ensure precise targeting and alignment, IGRT employs real-time imaging methods, such as CT scans or X-rays, to confirm the tumor's location before each radiation therapy session.

Stereotactic radiosurgery (SRS) or stereotactic body radiation therapy (SBRT): Using cutting-edge imaging and treatment planning tools, SBRT and SRS apply high doses of radiation to tiny, well-defined tumors or metastases in a limited number of treatment sessions, usually one to five.

2. Physical therapy: The process of brachytherapy, sometimes referred to as internal radiation treatment, involves injecting radioactive sources—such as pellets or seeds—directly into or close to the tumor site. The radioactive sources minimize radiation exposure to the surrounding healthy tissues while delivering a high dose of radiation to the tumor. Brachytherapy can be utilized for breast, cervical, or prostate cancer, either by itself or in conjunction with EBRT.

Thoughts Regarding Radiation Therapy:
1. Planning for Treatment: Patients go through a thorough treatment planning procedure before starting radiation therapy, which may involve imaging tests to properly characterize the tumor volume and surrounding anatomy, such as CT or MRI

scans. Together, medical physicists, dosimetrists, and radiation oncologists create a customized treatment plan that minimizes radiation exposure to healthy tissues while optimizing tumor control.

2. Diffusion: In order to maximize the efficiency of radiation therapy in killing cancer cells, radiation therapy is generally administered in many treatment sessions, or fractions, spread over several weeks. This allows healthy tissues to mend and recuperate in between treatments. Tumor type, size, location, and patient-specific characteristics are among the parameters that influence the total radiation dosage and the number of treatment fractions.

3. Adverse Impacts: Both short-term and long-term adverse effects from radiation therapy are possible, and they can differ based on the tumor's location and kind, the method of treatment, and the specifics of each patient. Acute adverse effects that are

frequently seen include tiredness, nausea, skin irritation or redness, and transient hair loss (in the treated region).
Radiation-induced secondary malignancies, fibrosis (scarring) of the treated region, and harm to surrounding organs or tissues are examples of long-term negative effects.

4. Immobilization and Positioning of the Patient: Accurate radiation therapy administration and limiting movement during treatment sessions depend on precise patient placement and immobilization. During the course of therapy, immobilization equipment like body frames, masks, or molds might be utilized to guarantee consistent posture and alignment.

5. After Care: Patients see their radiation oncologist on a regular basis after completing radiation therapy to discuss any unmet supportive care requirements, check treatment response, and evaluate for side effects or problems. Periodically, imaging examinations, including CT or PET scans, can be carried out to assess tumor response and disease progression.

Targeted and Immunotherapy

Targeted Therapy: Precision Medicine Approach

Targeted therapy is a cutting-edge method of treating cancer that focuses on locating and disrupting particular molecular targets necessary for the development and survival of cancer cells. Targeted therapy seeks to specifically target cancer cells while preserving healthy cells, reducing side effects, and enhancing treatment outcomes. This is in contrast to standard chemotherapy, which can impact both diseased and healthy cells. In this part, we shall examine the fundamentals, workings, and therapeutic uses of targeted therapy in the management of cancer.

Targeted Therapy Principles:
1. Molecular Mitigation: Finding certain molecular targets—such as proteins, enzymes, or genetic mutations—that are essential to the development and survival of cancer cells is the first step in targeted treatment. These targets could be connected to important signaling cascades, cell cycle control, angiogenesis (the creation of blood vessels), or processes for DNA repair.

2. Customized Care: Precision medicine, which acknowledges that every patient's cancer is different and may react differently to treatment depending on specific genetic mutations or molecular profiles, provides the foundation for targeted therapy. Through molecular testing, oncologists may determine the molecular profile of a patient's tumor and then customize treatment plans to specifically target genetic abnormalities or biomarkers that are responsible for the growth of cancer.

3. Medicine Design Rationale: Drugs used in targeted treatment are made to specifically inhibit or stop the activity of particular molecular targets that are thought to have a role in the initiation and spread of cancer. These medications are frequently monoclonal antibodies or tiny compounds that have the ability to enter cancer cells and disrupt biological processes necessary for tumor development or oncogenic signaling pathways.

Targeted Therapy Mechanisms:
1. Inhibition of Signal Transduction:
Inhibiting important signaling pathways involved in cancer cell survival, growth, and metastasis is how many targeted treatment medications function. Drugs that target pathways such as vascular endothelial growth factor (VEGF), human epidermal

growth factor receptor 2 (HER2), or the epidermal growth factor receptor (EGFR) can interfere with signaling cascades that encourage angiogenesis and tumor development.

2. Inhibition of Angiogenesis: The process of blood vessel development, which is necessary for tumor growth and metastasis, is the target of angiogenesis inhibitors. Angiogenesis inhibitors can disrupt tumor blood supply and limit tumor development by blocking angiogenic signaling pathways or directly targeting vascular endothelial growth factor (VEGF) or its receptors.

3. Apoptosis Induction: By focusing on certain proteins or pathways necessary for cell viability, some targeted treatment medications cause cancer cells to undergo programmed cell death, or apoptosis. For instance, by interfering with anti-apoptotic signaling pathways, inhibitors of the B-cell lymphoma 2 (BCL-2) protein family can induce apoptosis in cancer cells.

4. Immune Adjustment: By focusing on immunological checkpoint proteins that control T-cell activity, such as cytotoxic T-lymphocyte-associated protein 4 (CTLA-4) and programmed cell death protein 1 (PD-1), targeted therapy medications can also modify the immune response to cancer. In certain cancer types, immune checkpoint inhibitors can improve anti-tumor immune responses and encourage tumor regression.

Medicinal Uses of Targeted Treatment:
1. EGFR Inhibitors: EGFR-mutant non-small cell lung cancer (NSCLC), colorectal cancer, and head and neck cancer are treated with EGFR inhibitors such as gefitinib, erlotinib, and cetuximab. These medications inhibit the function of EGFR, a receptor tyrosine kinase linked to the development and spread of tumors.

2. HER2 Inhibitors: HER2-positive breast cancer and HER2-positive gastric or gastroesophageal junction cancer are treated with HER2 inhibitors, which include trastuzumab, pertuzumab, and ado-trastuzumab emtansine (T-DM1). These medications target HER2, a tyrosine kinase receptor that is overexpressed in several cancer types.

3. Inhibitors of MEK and BRAF: BRAF-mutant melanoma and BRAF-mutant non-small cell lung cancer (NSCLC) are treated with BRAF and MEK inhibitors, such as trametinib, dabrafenib, and vemurafenib. These medications target the dysregulated BRAF-MEK-ERK signaling pathway seen in tumors with BRAF mutations.

4. Inhibitors of PARP: BRCA-mutant ovarian cancer, breast cancer, and prostate cancer are treated with PARP inhibitors such as olaparib, rucaparib, and niraparib. These medications target the enzyme poly

(ADP-ribose) polymerase (PARP), which is involved in DNA repair and causes synthetic lethality in cancer cells lacking DNA repair machinery.

5. Inhibitors of Immune Checkpoints: Renal cell carcinoma, non-small cell lung cancer (NSCLC), and melanoma are among the cancers that are treated with immune checkpoint inhibitors like pembrolizumab, nivolumab, and ipilimumab. By inhibiting immunological checkpoint proteins like CTLA-4 or PD-1, these medications strengthen anti-tumor immune responses and enable the immune system to target cancer cells.

Attention to Detail in Targeted Therapy:
1. Molecular Characterization: Finding therapeutically useful genetic alterations or biomarkers that may be addressed with certain targeted treatment medications requires molecular profiling of the tumor. Molecular testing can assist in direct

treatment decisions and improve patient outcomes. Examples of such testing include polymerase chain reaction (PCR) and next-generation sequencing (NGS).

2. The Resistance to Drugs: Over time, cancer cells may become resistant to medications used in targeted therapy, which might result in the development of the illness and treatment failure. The development of next-generation inhibitors, combination therapy techniques, or focusing on alternative signaling pathways linked to cancer growth and survival are some strategies to combat drug resistance.

3. Impaired Impacts: Despite being typically less toxic than standard chemotherapy, targeted treatment medications can nonetheless have side effects such as skin rash, diarrhea, hypertension, and heart damage. Minimizing treatment-related morbidity and enhancing quality of life require close patient monitoring for adverse effects and prompt action.

4. Cost and Access: The cost of targeted therapy medications may be prohibitive, and some circumstances, such as insurance coverage, healthcare inequities, and the accessibility of certain medicines in particular locations or healthcare settings, may restrict access to these treatments. Making targeted therapy medications more accessible, affordable, and fairly distributed is essential to guaranteeing that all patients may take advantage of these cutting-edge therapeutic modalities.

Immunotherapy: Harnessing the Body's Immune System

Utilizing the body's immune system to identify, target, and eradicate cancer cells, immunotherapy is a novel method of cancer treatment. Instead of going after cancer cells directly like surgery, chemotherapy, or radiation therapy, immunotherapy works by improving or modifying the immune response so that cancer cells are more easily identified and attacked while normal tissues are spared. In this part, we shall examine the fundamentals, workings, therapeutic uses, and issues surrounding immunotherapy in the treatment of cancer.

The Immunotherapy Principles:
1. Immune Response Enhancement: By stimulating or increasing immune cells, such as T cells, natural killer (NK) cells, or dendritic cells, to more efficiently identify and destroy cancer cells, immunotherapy

seeks to improve the body's immunological response to cancer.

2. Getting Rid of Immune Evasion:

Through a variety of strategies, including the downregulation of major histocompatibility complex (MHC) molecules, the upregulation of immune checkpoint proteins (like PD-L1, CTLA-4), or the secretion of immunosuppressive factors (like TGF-β, IL-10), cancer cells can avoid the immune system's recognition and destruction. Restoring anti-tumor immunity and defeating immune evasion mechanisms are the goals of immunotherapy therapies.

3. Creating Immune Memory: Long-lasting immunological memory against cancer may be induced by immunotherapy, which might result in persistent anti-tumor immunity and defense against disease spread or recurrence.

The mechanisms of immunotherapy:
1. Inhibition of Immune Checkpoint:
Immune checkpoint inhibitors (ICIs) are a class of immunotherapy medications that specifically target immune checkpoint proteins that are known to downregulate T cell activity and inhibit anti-tumor immune responses. Examples of these proteins include cytotoxic T-lymphocyte-associated protein 4 (CTLA-4), programmed cell death protein 1 (PD-1), and programmed death ligand 1 (PD-L1). ICIs effectively release the immune system to target cancer cells by obstructing immunological checkpoint pathways.

2. CAR-T Cell Therapy: This type of treatment uses a patient's own T cells to express chimeric antigen receptors (CARs), which are artificial receptors made to detect certain antigens expressed on cancer cells. Tumor regression and remission can result from CAR-T cells' ability to identify and eliminate cancer cells that express the target antigen after they have been reinfused into the patient.

3. The use of monoclonal antibodies
Monoclonal antibodies are created in laboratories with the primary purpose of targeting antigens expressed in cancer cells. These antibodies have the ability to attach directly to cancer cells, which can promote the death of cancer cells by complement-mediated cytotoxicity, antibody-dependent cellular cytotoxicity (ADCC), or apoptosis induction.

4. Vaccines against cancer: By exposing immune cells like T cells or dendritic cells to tumor-specific antigens or peptides, cancer vaccines seek to activate the immune system to identify and combat cancer cells. Cancer vaccines can be created to specifically target neoantigens—antigens formed from mutations unique to cancer—or tumor-associated antigens.

Medical Uses of Immunotherapy:

1. PD-1/PD-L1 Inhibitors: PD-1/PD-L1 inhibitors are used to treat a variety of cancers, including bladder cancer, melanoma, renal cell carcinoma, non-small cell lung cancer (NSCLC), and Hodgkin lymphoma. Examples of these inhibitors include pembrolizumab, nivolumab, and atezolizumab. By preventing T cells' PD-1 on T cells from interacting with cancer cells' PD-L1, these medications restore T cell-mediated anti-tumor immunity.

2. CTLA-4 Inhibitors: Melanoma and other malignancies are treated with CTLA-4 inhibitors, such as ipilimumab. Through the inhibition of CTLA-4, an anti-tumor immune response that controls T cell activation and proliferation, CTLA-4 inhibitors facilitate tumor regression.

3. CAR-T Cell Therapy: In the treatment of several hematological malignancies, including diffuse large B-cell lymphoma

(DLBCL), multiple myeloma, and acute lymphoblastic leukemia (ALL), CAR-T cell therapy has demonstrated exceptional clinical success. Axiscarta (Yescarta) and Tisagenlecleucel (Kymriah) are two examples of CAR-T cell treatments that have received FDA approval.

4. Antibodies that are monoclonal: Trastuzumab (HER2/neu), rituximab (CD20), and cetuximab (EGFR) are examples of monoclonal antibodies that target particular antigens and are used to treat HER2-positive breast cancer, B-cell lymphomas, and head and neck cancer, respectively. These antibodies have the ability to inhibit signaling pathways necessary for cancer cell survival or cause antibody-dependent cellular cytotoxicity (ADCC).

Immunotherapy Considerations

1. IrAEs, or immune-related adverse events: Due to dysregulated immune activation against normal tissues, immunotherapy might result in immune-related adverse events (irAEs). Skin rash, colitis, pneumonitis, hepatitis, thyroid dysfunction, or endocrine abnormalities are examples of common adverse events (irAEs). Improving patient outcomes and reducing treatment-related morbidity require early identification and management of irAEs.

2. Analysis of Response: Immunotherapy may result in unusual response patterns, such as delayed responses or pseudoprogression, which may need to be carefully distinguished from disease progression by clinical surveillance and rigorous radiological examination. To precisely evaluate the response to immunotherapy, immune-related response assessment criteria in solid tumors (iRECIST) or immune-related response criteria (irRC) have been developed.

3. Biomarker Testing: Biomarker testing, such as determining the status of microsatellite instability (MSI), tumor mutational burden (TMB), or PD-L1 expression levels, may help determine which patients are most likely to benefit from immunotherapy and direct treatment choices. Additionally, prognosis and responsiveness to certain immunotherapy medicines or combination treatments can be predicted by biomarker testing. Combination therapies, including immunotherapy and chemotherapy, immunotherapy and targeted therapy, or dual checkpoint blockade (e.g., PD-1/PD-L1 plus CTLA-4 inhibitors), are being researched to improve treatment efficacy and address resistance mechanisms in cancer. Combinatorial strategies have the potential to improve clinical outcomes and strengthen anti-tumor immune responses in concert.

Combination Therapies and Clinical Trials

Combination treatments, which combine immunotherapy and targeted therapy, have shown promise in the treatment of cancer. They can overcome resistance mechanisms, increase therapeutic effectiveness, and improve patient outcomes. These novel strategies make use of the complementary mechanisms of action of immunotherapeutic drugs and targeted medicines to provide combined actions against cancer cells. The justification for combination therapy, current clinical studies, and possible ramifications for cancer care will all be covered in this section.

Justification for Combination Treatments:

1. Collaborative Benefits: The unique modes of action of targeted therapy and immunotherapy can work together to strengthen anti-tumor immune responses and increase therapeutic results. By upregulating tumor antigen expression or altering the tumor microenvironment, for instance, targeted medicines may sensitize cancer cells to immune-mediated death and increase the effectiveness of immunotherapy.

2. Getting Past Resistance: Through a variety of methods, including genetic changes, adaptive immune evasion, or the activation of compensatory signaling pathways, cancer cells can become resistant to single-agent therapy. Patients with advanced or resistant malignancies may benefit from combination therapy that targets many immunological checkpoints or signaling pathways in order to overcome resistance mechanisms and produce more robust responses.

3. Maximizing the Order of Treatment:

The order in which immunotherapy and targeted therapy are given can affect the course of treatment and how well patients respond. Targeted treatment can be administered sequentially or concurrently with immunotherapy, or vice versa, to take advantage of the special vulnerabilities present in cancer cells and optimize therapeutic efficacy while reducing toxicity.

Combination Therapy Examples:

1. Dual Checkpoint Blockade: Combining immune checkpoint inhibitors that target distinct immune checkpoints, such as cytotoxic T-lymphocyte-associated protein 4 (CTLA-4) and programmed cell death protein 1 (PD-1) has been shown to have synergistic effects in improving clinical outcomes and anti-tumor immune responses in a variety of cancer types, including renal cell carcinoma, melanoma, and non-small cell lung cancer (NSCLC).

2. Combinations of Targeted Therapy and Immunotherapy: When immunotherapy is combined with targeted agents—such as EGFR inhibitors for non-small cell lung cancer (NSCLC) or BRAF or MEK inhibitors for melanoma—that alter particular signaling pathways linked to the growth and survival of cancer, the combination has been shown to be more effective and to prolong progression-free survival longer than when the agents are used alone.

3. Combotherapy and Immunotherapy Sets: Chemotherapy medications can influence immune cell populations, stimulate the release of tumor antigens, or interfere with immune suppressive systems in the tumor microenvironment to produce immunomodulatory effects. Combination treatments that include immunotherapy and chemotherapy have demonstrated encouraging outcomes in triple-negative breast cancer, ovarian cancer, and bladder cancer, among other disease types.

Clinical Trials Underway:

First/Second Phase Trials: Patients with advanced or resistant malignancies are participating in phase I and II clinical studies to assess the safety, tolerability, and potential effectiveness of innovative combination treatments. In order to identify patient populations most likely to benefit from combination therapy and to define the ideal treatment regimen, these trials frequently incorporate expansion cohorts and dosage escalation.

2. Trials for Phase III: Phase III clinical trials are intended to evaluate, in sizable patient populations, the safety and effectiveness of combination medicines in comparison to standard-of-care or single-agent therapies. The purpose of these studies is to get regulatory permission for the use of combination treatments in clinical practice and to establish them as routine treatment alternatives.

3. Trials Driven by Biomarkers: Clinical trials that are driven by biomarkers are investigating how to identify individuals who are most likely to benefit from combination therapy by using predictive biomarkers such as tumor mutational burden (TMB), microsatellite instability (MSI), or immune cell infiltration. Based on unique tumor biology and immunological profiles, these trials seek to enhance patient outcomes and tailor treatment modalities.

Repercussions for Cancer Treatment:
1. Precision Medicine: Combination treatments mark a paradigm shift in cancer therapy toward precision medicine, wherein patient-specific variables and the molecular features of the tumor inform treatment choices. Oncologists can customize treatment plans to target certain

vulnerabilities of cancer cells and maximize therapeutic efficacy by combining targeted therapy with immunotherapy.

2. Long-Term Survival: By enhancing long-term survival results and producing persistent responses in patients with advanced or metastatic illnesses, combination treatments hold the potential to revolutionize the delivery of cancer therapy. For patients with few treatment options and a dismal prognosis, these novel methods of treatment provide new hope by combining the synergistic benefits of immunotherapy and targeted therapy.

3. Goals for the Future: Research endeavors are presently concentrated on the identification of creative combination methods, the clarification of fundamental processes of synergy and resistance, and the investigation of novel therapeutic modalities, including tumor vaccines, CAR-T cell therapy, and oncolytic viruses. These developments have the potential to increase treatment results and broaden the range of available cancer treatments.

Part III: Integrative Approaches

Mind-Body Connection

Understanding the Mind-Body Connection

The complex interaction that exists between our ideas, feelings, beliefs, and physical health is known as the "mind-body connection." It emphasizes how profoundly our emotional and mental moods may affect our physical health and vice versa. Enhancing general health and wellbeing might result from acknowledging and fostering this relationship. This article will discuss the idea of the mind-body link, how it affects health, and practical methods for maximizing its effects.

The Impact of Emotions and Thoughts on Health

Psychoneuroimmunology research has shown strong evidence of the immune system, neurological system, and brain communicating with each other in both directions. Our ideas, beliefs, and feelings have a direct effect on how our hormone balance, immune system, and other physiological systems work. Chronic stress, for instance, has been connected to immunological suppression, inflammation, and heightened vulnerability to disease, whereas happy, thankful, and optimistic feelings can strengthen the immune system and encourage recovery.

Stress's Function:

Stress may have a significant impact on our physical health and well-being, whether it is acute or chronic. Stress triggers a complicated physiological reaction in our bodies called the stress response, sometimes referred to as the "fight-or-flight" response. This reaction includes the production of stress hormones, including cortisol and adrenaline. Although this reaction is short-term adaptive, long-term stress can dysregulate the stress response system, which can have negative consequences on immune system performance, digestion, mental health, and cardiovascular health.

Impacts of Meditation and Mindfulness: Deep breathing exercises, yoga, and other mindfulness techniques have been demonstrated to reduce stress, increase relaxation, and foster a sense of inner calm and wellbeing. Being mindful entails focusing on the here and now with acceptance, curiosity, and openness—without passing judgment. People can improve emotional resilience, self-awareness, and compassion while lowering stress, anxiety, and rumination by practicing mindfulness.

The Brain-Gut Axis:
Recent studies have brought attention to the role that the gut-brain axis plays in regulating the mind-body relationship. The enteric nervous system, a sophisticated network of neurons found in the stomach that is sometimes referred to as the "second brain," is in bidirectional communication with the central nervous system through the vagus nerve. The billions of bacteria and other microorganisms that make up the gut microbiota are essential for controlling mood, behavior, and brain function because they produce hormones, neurotransmitters, and inflammatory mediators.

Techniques to Strengthen the Mind-Body Bond:
Mindfulness Techniques: To encourage relaxation, lower stress levels, and improve general well-being, incorporate mindfulness techniques into your daily routine. These techniques include yoga, tai chi, meditation, and deep breathing exercises.

Good Lifestyle Practices: Developing a healthy lifestyle that incorporates stress reduction strategies, a balanced diet, regular exercise, and enough sleep can enhance the mind-body connection and improve both physical and mental well-being.

Emotional Expression: Seek out social assistance when necessary, acknowledge and analyze your emotions, and build good relationships with others to engage in healthy emotional expression.

Self-Care: Make time for self-care activities that feed your mind, body, and soul. Some examples of these include taking up a hobby, going on a nature walk, practicing gratitude, and establishing boundaries to safeguard your energy and overall wellbeing.

Professional Support: To improve the mind-body connection and address particular health issues, seek the advice, support, and customized solutions of mental health specialists, counselors, or holistic practitioners.

Stress Reduction Techniques

Stress has become a common problem, impacting both mental and physical health in today's fast-paced environment. Prolonged stress affects not just our mental health but also our physical health, which makes a number of health issues more likely to arise. Knowing the relationship between the mind and body can help us integrate methods that support both the physical and mental components of well-being to successfully manage stress. We'll look at a few practical stress-reduction strategies in this part that support mental and physical balance.

1. Meditation with mindfulness:

Practicing mindfulness meditation entails developing present-moment awareness by paying attention, without passing judgment, to the breath, physical sensations, thoughts, and emotions. Regular mindfulness meditation practice can help promote relaxation, emotional resilience, and general well-being while lowering stress, anxiety, and rumination. Studies have demonstrated that mindfulness-based therapies can result in both structural and functional alterations in the brain that are linked to enhanced stress management and emotional control.

2. Practices for Deep Breathing:

Exercises involving deep breathing, such as diaphragmatic breathing or belly breathing, entail taking slow, deep breaths with the nose to fill the lungs, then gently letting go of the air through the mouth to enable the abdomen to rise and fall with each breath. By inducing the parasympathetic nervous system and triggering the body's relaxation response, deep breathing lowers the physiological effects of stress, including elevated blood pressure, heart rate, and tense muscles. Spending a few minutes each day doing deep breathing exercises will help you become more relaxed, peaceful, and able to think clearly.

3. The gradual relaxation of muscles (PMR):

A method known as progressive muscle relaxation involves methodically tensing and releasing various body muscular groups, working your way up to the head from the feet. PMR eases symptoms of stress-related muscular tension and discomfort by deliberately tensing and releasing muscle tension. It also decreases muscle stiffness and soreness. People who regularly practice PMR can learn to release tension from their bodies and become more aware of the bodily signs of stress.

4. Assisted Visualization and Imagery:

Using techniques such as guided imagery and visualization, one may mentally picture settings or scenarios that are quiet, relaxing, and elicit good feelings and sensations, such as a calm beach, lush forest, or placid garden. Guided imagery can lower stress hormone levels, induce a relaxation response in the body, and foster emotions of inner calm and well-being by stimulating the senses and the imagination. Scripts or recordings for guided imagery can be used to lead people through visualizations suited to their requirements and preferences.

5. Tai Chi and Yoga:

Yoga and Tai Chi are mind-body exercises that integrate breathing techniques, physical postures, and meditation to enhance awareness, flexibility, and relaxation. In order to promote inner balance and harmony, these age-old techniques place a strong emphasis on mindful movement, breath awareness, and present-moment awareness. Regular yoga and tai chi practice can help build a stronger bond between the mind and body, lower stress, increase physical fitness, and improve mental clarity.

6. Expressive Writing and Journaling: Expressive writing and journaling offer a creative avenue for managing feelings, investigating ideas, and discovering stresses and triggers. People can acquire clarity about their experiences and feelings, let go of pent-up emotions, and create healthy coping mechanisms for stress management by writing down their thoughts and feelings. In addition to encouraging self-reflection, appreciation, and goal-setting, journaling may also help with self-empowerment and resilience.

Meditation and Mindfulness Principles:
In contemplative practices like mindfulness and meditation, the focus is on purposefully bringing attention to the present moment with openness, curiosity, and nonjudgmental awareness. Through these techniques, people can develop a feeling of inner calm, clarity, and acceptance by learning to notice their thoughts, emotions, physical sensations, and external environment without attachment or aversion. Through the practice of attentional concentration and mindfulness, people may improve their ability to regulate their emotions, become more resilient to stress, and strengthen their bonds with both the outside world and themselves.

Advantages of Mindfulness and Meditation:
1. "Reduction of Stress Reducing tension and promoting relaxation is one of the most well-established effects of mindfulness and meditation. Regular meditation and

mindfulness practice can help people better handle everyday pressures, increase resilience to adversity, and improve general well-being by triggering the body's relaxation response and regulating stress hormone levels.

2. Emotional Regulation: Through the cultivation of increased awareness of thoughts, emotions, and habitual patterns of reaction, mindfulness and meditation techniques help people respond to difficult situations with more composure and clarity. Mindfulness cultivates emotional resilience, self-compassion, and pleasant mood states by encouraging a non-reactive, non-judgmental attitude toward internal feelings, such as fear, rage, or grief.

3. Enhanced Focus and Cognitive Abilities: Mindfulness Training attentional control, cognitive flexibility, and working memory capacity are three ways that meditation improves cognitive performance. People

can enhance their ability to concentrate, focus, and complete cognitive tasks in a variety of contexts, including academic, professional, and artistic endeavors, by engaging in practices of sustaining attention to the present moment and refocusing attention from distractions.

4. Better Self-Awareness and Understanding: By shedding light on the ingrained thought, emotion, and behavior patterns that influence our subjective perception of reality, mindfulness and meditation techniques help us become more self-aware. People can learn more about the nature of their minds by engaging in introspection and self-reflection, which can reveal ingrained prejudices, training, and beliefs that affect how they see the world and behave. Increased self-awareness promotes self-discovery, personal development, and alignment with goals and basic beliefs.

Meditation and Mindfulness Techniques

The practices of mindfulness and meditation have grown in popularity as useful strategies for enhancing mental clarity, emotional balance, and general well-being in our fast-paced, modern society. Meditation and mindfulness techniques, which have their roots in age-old contemplative traditions, provide significant insights into the mind-body connection and help us comprehend the complex relationship that exists between our ideas, emotions, and bodily sensations. This section will examine the tenets, advantages, and methods of mindfulness and meditation for fostering a positive mind-body connection.

Meditation and Mindfulness Principles:
In contemplative practices like mindfulness and meditation, the focus is on purposefully bringing attention to the present moment with openness, curiosity, and nonjudgmental awareness. Through these techniques, people can develop a feeling of inner calm, clarity, and acceptance by learning to notice their thoughts, emotions, physical sensations, and external environment without attachment or aversion. Through the practice of attentional concentration and mindfulness, people may improve their ability to regulate their emotions, become more resilient to stress, and strengthen their bonds with both the outside world and themselves.

Advantages of Mindfulness and Meditation:
1. Reduction of Stress Reducing tension and promoting relaxation is one of the most well-established effects of mindfulness and meditation. Regular meditation and

mindfulness practice can help people better handle everyday pressures, increase resilience to adversity, and improve general well-being by triggering the body's relaxation response and regulating stress hormone levels.

2. Emotional Regulation: Through the cultivation of increased awareness of thoughts, emotions, and habitual patterns of reaction, mindfulness and meditation techniques help people respond to difficult situations with more composure and clarity. Mindfulness cultivates emotional resilience, self-compassion, and pleasant mood states by encouraging a non-reactive, non-judgmental attitude toward internal feelings, such as fear, rage, or grief.

3. Enhanced Focus and Cognitive Abilities: Mindfulness Training attentional control, cognitive flexibility, and working memory capacity are three ways that meditation improves cognitive performance.

People can enhance their ability to concentrate, focus, and complete cognitive tasks in a variety of contexts, including academic, professional, and artistic endeavors, by engaging in practices of sustaining attention to the present moment and refocusing attention from distractions.

4. Better Self-Awareness and Understanding: By shedding light on the ingrained thought, emotion, and behavior patterns that influence our subjective perception of reality, mindfulness and meditation techniques help us become more self-aware. People can learn more about the nature of their minds by engaging in introspection and self-reflection, which can reveal ingrained prejudices, training, and beliefs that affect how they see the world and behave. Increased self-awareness promotes self-discovery, personal development, and alignment with goals and basic beliefs.

1. Meditation with Focused Attention and Concentration: This technique involves concentrating attention on only one thing at a time, such as the breath, a mantra, or a picture. To foster prolonged attention and mental stability, the selected item is gently brought back into focus if the mind strays.

2. Open Monitoring (Cognitive) Practice: Non-judgmental awareness of one's thoughts, feelings, physical sensations, and environmental stimuli is all part of this practice. The whole field of consciousness is brought into focus rather than just one particular thing, which encourages an open-minded and welcoming attitude toward whatever comes up.

3. Body Scan Meditation: This technique involves methodically focusing attention on various body parts, beginning with the toes and working your way up to the head. Body scan meditation encourages relaxation, somatic awareness, and embodiment by developing an awareness of one's own body feelings and relieving tension or discomfort.

4. Meditating while strolling: Walking meditation combines mindfulness with physical exercise, enabling participants to walk slowly and deliberately while cultivating awareness of their breath, surroundings, and bodily sensations. A sense of presence, groundedness, and connection to the land are fostered by focusing attention on the sensations of walking with each stride.

Therapy

Herbal Remedies and Supplements

Herbal treatments and supplements are important tools in the holistic health and therapy fields for promoting general wellbeing and managing a range of medical disorders. Herbal treatments and supplements, which have their roots in ancient healing traditions and are supported by contemporary scientific study, provide a natural substitute for conventional drugs. These alternatives often have fewer side effects and emphasize the body's natural healing processes. We will examine the advantages, factors to take into account, and therapeutic uses of herbal treatments and supplements as we dig into the field of herbal therapy.

Comprehending Herbal Medicine:

Herbal therapy, often referred to as botanical medicine or herbalism, is the use of plants and products derived from plants to cure, prevent, or mitigate medical diseases. This age-old therapeutic technique, which promotes health and vitality by using the medicinal qualities of herbs, roots, leaves, flowers, and other botanicals, has been used for ages in civilizations all over the world. Herbal medicines can have a variety of therapeutic effects and modalities of administration since they are commonly prepared as teas, tinctures, capsules, powders, or topical ointments.

Advantages of Supplements and Herbal Remedies:
1. Healing Naturally: Strong bioactive chemicals, antioxidants, vitamins, and minerals that assist the body's natural healing processes are found in herbal treatments and supplements, which capitalize on the healing power of nature.

Herbal medications, in contrast to manufactured pharmaceuticals, come from natural sources and can contain a wide variety of complex phytochemicals that combine to support health and vitality.

2. Holistic Approach: Rather than focusing only on treating symptoms, herbal therapy promotes a holistic approach to health and wellbeing, addressing the underlying causes of sickness and imbalances. Herbal medicines improve overall vitality and help restore equilibrium to the body's systems, promoting physical, mental, and emotional well-being.

3. Less Adverse Effects: Supplements and herbal medicines are typically thought to be safer, kinder, and less likely to cause negative effects than synthetic medications. Herbal remedies can provide effective treatment for medical ailments without having negative side effects or upsetting the body's natural equilibrium when taken as directed by a skilled practitioner.

4. Personalized Attention: Herbal therapy enables customized treatment plans based on the specific constitution, health issues, and preferences of the patient. When choosing herbal medicines, herbalists and holistic practitioners consider a variety of criteria, including body type, constitution, lifestyle, and environmental effects. This ensures that each patient receives individualized and comprehensive care for the best possible therapeutic results.

Typical Supplements and Herbal Remedies:

1. Curcuma longa, or turmeric: Turmeric, well-known for its strong anti-inflammatory and antioxidant qualities, has been used in traditional medicine to assist digestion, lessen inflammation, ease pain, and enhance general health. The key ingredient in turmeric, curcumin, has been the subject of much research into its potential treatment benefits for a range of illnesses, including neurological diseases, cardiovascular disease, and arthritis.

2. Zingiber officinale, or ginger: Thanks to its well-known digestive, anti-nausea, and anti-inflammatory qualities, ginger is often used as a treatment for menstrual cramps, gastrointestinal discomfort, and motion sickness. Gingerols, the bioactive chemicals found in ginger, work as analgesics and anti-inflammatory agents by blocking pro-inflammatory cytokines and pain-sensing enzymes.

Echinacea purpurea, or Echinacea: Echinacea is widely used to boost immunity and strengthen defenses against illnesses, including the flu and colds. Bioactive substances found in this plant, such as polysaccharides and alkylamides, boost immune system function, boost the formation of antibodies, and shorten the length and intensity of respiratory infections.

4. Withania somnifera, or Ashwagandha: In Ayurvedic medicine, ashwagandha is an adaptogenic herb that is used to boost adrenal function, increase energy, and foster resistance to stress. The active ingredients in ashwagandha, called withanolides, help the body adjust to stress and maintain homeostasis by regulating cortisol levels and modulating the hypothalamic-pituitary-adrenal (HPA) axis.

5. Fatty Acids Omega-3: Omega-3 fatty acids have been demonstrated to enhance cardiovascular health, cognitive function, mood stability, and inflammatory balance. They are present in fatty fish (such as salmon, mackerel, and sardines), flaxseeds, chia seeds, and walnuts. Omega-3 fatty acid supplements may assist in blood pressure reduction, cholesterol improvement, inflammation reduction, and brain health support.

Thoughts on Herbal Therapy:
1. Safety and Quality: To guarantee purity, potency, and safety, choose premium products from reliable producers when selecting herbal remedies and supplements. To ensure quality and authenticity, look for organic ingredients, standardized extracts, and independent testing.

2. Interaction with Medications: Supplements and herbal remedies may have interactions with some medications that could compromise their safety or effectiveness. It's crucial to speak with a licensed healthcare professional, especially if you take prescription drugs, in order to prevent any negative effects or drug interactions.

3. Personal hypersensitivity: Although most people find herbal remedies to be safe, certain people may experience allergies or sensitivities. It is best to start with a modest dose and keep an eye out for any sensitivities or negative responses. In the event that you encounter any peculiar symptoms, stop using the product and seek medical advice.

4. A Practitioner Consultation: It is best to use herbal therapy under the supervision of a trained professional, such as an integrative medicine physician, a naturopathic physician, or a licensed herbalist. These medical specialists may offer tailored advice, monitoring, and dosage guidance to guarantee the safe and efficient use of supplements and herbal medicines.

Part IV: Nutrition and Wellness

Anti-Cancer Diet and Nutrition

Key Nutrients for Cancer Prevention

In order to prevent cancer and maintain general health, diet and nutrition are very important. Studies indicate that some foods and dietary habits may mitigate the development of cancer by bolstering the body's innate defensive systems, enhancing cellular well-being, and diminishing inflammation. We'll go over important nutrients that have been linked to cancer prevention in our guide to an anti-cancer diet, along with advice on how to include them in your regular meals.

1. Antioxidants:

Antioxidants are substances that aid in the neutralization of dangerous free radicals, which can cause damage to DNA and cells and aid in the emergence of cancer. You can lower your risk of cancer and defend against oxidative stress by including foods high in antioxidants in your diet. Typical antioxidants include the following:

Vitamin C: Found in broccoli, bell peppers, strawberries, kiwis, and citrus fruits.
Vitamin E: Contains nuts, seeds, spinach, and cereals that have been fortified.
- Beta-carotene: Found in kale, spinach, carrots, sweet potatoes, and apricots.
Selenium: It occurs in whole grains, shellfish, lean meats, and Brazil nuts.

2. Phytochemicals

Foods derived from plants include bioactive substances called phytochemicals, which have been demonstrated to have anti-cancer effects. These substances work through a variety of pathways, such as anti-inflammatory, anti-carcinogenic, and antioxidant ones. Among the noteworthy phytochemicals are:

Flavonoids: present in red wine, tea, fruits, and vegetables. Quercetin, kaempferol, and catechins are a few examples.
Isoflavones are present in legumes, tofu, soybeans, and tempeh. Daidzein and genistein are two examples.
Indoles: Included in cruciferous vegetables, including Brussels sprouts, broccoli, cabbage, and cauliflower. Indole-3-carbinol and sulforaphane are two examples.

3. Tissue:

The consumption of dietary fiber is essential for maintaining intestinal health, controlling bowel motions, and lowering the risk of colorectal cancer. Consuming a diet high in fiber can help increase the excretion of carcinogens, avoid constipation, and maintain a healthy gut flora. Dietary fiber sources include:

Whole grains: Include whole wheat, quinoa, barley, oats, and brown rice.
Legumes: Including peas, beans, lentils, and chickpeas.
Vegetables and fruits: particularly leafy greens, apples, pears, berries, and other fruits with edible seeds or skins.

4. Fatty Acids Omega-3:

Essential fats with anti-inflammatory qualities and the potential to lower the risk of several cancer types are omega-3 fatty acids. Walnuts, hemp seeds, chia seeds, flaxseeds, and fatty fish all contain these good fats. Including foods high in omega-3 fatty acids in your diet can promote general health and help you keep your fatty acid balance in check.

5. Vegetables with a Crucifix:

Cruciferous vegetables are high in glucosinolates, which are sulfur-containing chemicals with shown anti-cancer properties. High quantities of fiber, vitamins, and minerals that promote general health are also present in these veggies. Broccoli, cauliflower, Brussels sprouts, kale, and cabbage are cruciferous vegetables.

6. Green Tea:

Polyphenols found in green tea, specifically catechins, have been researched for possible anti-cancer effects. Regular use of green tea has been linked to a lower chance of developing several malignancies, such as colorectal, prostate, and breast cancer. To optimize the health advantages of green tea, choose unsweetened varieties.

7. Vibrant Fruits and Vegetables:

A wide range of vitamins, minerals, antioxidants, and phytochemicals that promote general health and may help lower the risk of cancer are available when consuming a variety of colored fruits and vegetables. Eat as many different hues of the rainbow as possible, such as purple grapes, orange carrots, yellow bell peppers, red tomatoes, and green leafy vegetables. issues.

Sample Meal Plans and Recipes

Adopting a nutrient-dense, anti-cancer diet can help to promote general health and well-being while lowering the chance of cancer development. Organizing your meals to include a range of cancer-preventive foods can help you stay on top of your nutritional intake and maintain a balanced diet. Here are some sample menus and dishes that are meant to encourage good health and lower the risk of cancer.

Model Meal Schedule:
First Day:

Breakfast: overnight oats with sliced almonds, fresh berries, and honey drizzled on top.
herbal or green tea.

Lunch:
A salad made of quinoa, mixed greens, grilled chicken, cherry tomatoes, cucumber, and avocado.
Tahini and lemon dressing.

Snack: banana slices topped with Greek yogurt and cinnamon.

Supper:
Baked salmon served with sweet potatoes and roasted asparagus.
Broccoli cooked in olive oil and garlic.
roll made of whole grains.

Second Day:
Breakfast: Poached egg, sliced tomatoes, and mashed avocado on whole grain bread. squeezed orange juice right away.

Lunch: Turmeric, Kale, Carrots, and Celery in a Lentil Soup.
Grain crackers whole.

Snack: almond butter on apple slices.

Supper:
Tofu skewers grilled with onions, mushrooms, and bell peppers.
Quinoa pilaf topped with pine nuts and spinach.
A mixed-berry salad dressed with a balsamic dressing.

Instructions:
1. Dressing with Lemon-Tahini
Two teaspoons of fresh lemon juice 1/4 cup tahini

Two teaspoons of water and one minced
garlic clove
One teaspoon of maple syrup or honey
To taste, add salt and pepper.

Guidelines:
1. To make the tahini smooth and creamy,
combine the tahini, lemon juice, water,
garlic, honey or maple syrup, salt, and
pepper in a small bowl.
2. If necessary, add additional water to
adjust consistency.
3. Use as a dipping sauce for veggies or
drizzle over salads.

2. Turmeric and Kale Lentil Soup:
One cup of washed and drained green
lentils
One chopped onion, two diced carrots, and
two diced celery stalks
Three minced garlic cloves
One teaspoon of powdered turmeric
2 cups finely chopped kale 6 cups of
vegetable broth

Season with salt and pepper. Garnish with fresh parsley.

Guidelines:
1. Saute the onion, celery, carrots, and garlic in a big saucepan until they are tender.
2. Cook for a further minute after adding the turmeric powder.
3. Include the veggie broth and lentils. Once the lentils are soft, bring to a boil, lower the heat, and simmer for 20 to 25 minutes.
4. Add the chopped kale and simmer, stirring, until wilted, about 5 more minutes.
5. To taste, add salt and pepper for seasoning. Before serving, garnish with fresh parsley.

3. Tofu Skewers Grilled:
One block of extra-firm tofu that has been pressed and diced.
Two bell peppers, sliced into pieces.
One red onion, sliced into pieces
Eight to ten button mushrooms

30 minutes of water soaking for wooden skewers

Marinade:
One tablespoon sesame oil; two cloves of minced garlic 1/4 cup soy sauce or tamari
Two teaspoons of maple syrup and two tablespoons of rice vinegar
One teaspoon finely chopped ginger
To taste, add salt and pepper.

Guidelines:
1. Combine the marinade ingredients in a bowl.
2. Thread bell peppers, onions, mushrooms, and chunks of tofu onto skewers.
3. After setting the skewers in a shallow dish, cover them with marinade, twisting to ensure a uniform coating. Give it a minimum of half an hour to marinade.
4. Set the grill pan or grill to medium heat. Grill the skewers for five to seven minutes on each side, or until the veggies are soft and the tofu is gently browned.

Exercise and Physical Wellness

Benefits of Exercise for Cancer Patients

Physical fitness and exercise are essential components of everyone's overall health, even cancer sufferers. Even though receiving cancer treatment can be emotionally and physically taxing, patients can reap several advantages from including regular exercise in their regimen. This article will examine the benefits of exercise for cancer patients and emphasize how it may raise their standard of living.

1. Increased Physical Strength and Endurance: Cancer patients can see an increase in their physical strength and endurance by regularly exercising. Depending on one's capacities, physical activity can help counteract the weariness that cancer therapies frequently cause. Patients may see increases in stamina and ease in doing everyday duties by progressively increasing their exercise levels.

2. Lessened therapy negative effects: Research has indicated that exercise helps lessen a few of the typical negative effects of cancer therapy. For example, exercise helps lessen the intensity of nausea, exhaustion, and discomfort associated with chemotherapy. Exercise can also improve cardiovascular health, which can be harmed by some cancer therapies.

3. Enhanced Mental Health: Physical activity helps cancer patients stay physically well, but it also enhances their mental health. Frequent exercise releases endorphins, which are organic mood enhancers. This may lessen the tension, worry, and sadness that cancer patients frequently feel. Exercise also helps one feel in control of their body and empowered, which promotes a good outlook.

4. Enhanced immunological function:
Research indicates that physical activity has a favorable effect on the immunological system. Patients with cancer frequently have compromised immune systems as a result of their illness or the therapies they receive. Patients who exercise regularly may be able to boost their immune systems, which might enhance their general health and lower their risk of illness.

5. Weight Management and Body Composition: It is critical for cancer patients to maintain a healthy weight since it can have a favorable effect on their general well-being and the effectiveness of their therapy. Patients can better control their weight and enhance their body composition by combining a healthy diet and regular exercise. This may result in a more favorable reaction to therapy, a lower chance of problems, and higher self-esteem.

6. Improved Quality of Life: Cancer patients' quality of life may be considerably improved by exercise. Exercise can assist patients in regaining a sense of normality and control over their lives by strengthening their bodies, lowering the negative effects of therapy, enhancing mental health, and encouraging general health. Additionally, it can offer chances for assistance and social engagement, which can improve their wellbeing even more.

Safe and Efficient Exercise Protocols

Retaining physical well-being and general health depends heavily on exercise. It not only aids in weight management but also strengthens the heart, elevates mood, and promotes general wellbeing. Nonetheless, in order to optimize the advantages and reduce the chance of harm, it's critical to exercise properly and efficiently. We'll provide you with safe and practical workout tips in this post so you can include exercise in your daily routine and get the best results possible.

1. Speak with a healthcare expert: It's important to speak with a healthcare expert before beginning any fitness program, particularly if you have any underlying medical ailments or concerns. They are able to evaluate your present state of health and offer tailored advice according to your particular requirements and constraints.

2. Begin gently and gradually raise intensity: It's crucial to begin your exercises gently and gradually raise their intensity if you've never worked out before or if you've been inactive for a long time. This lowers the chance of harm and enables your body to adjust. Start with low-impact exercises like cycling, swimming, or walking, and as your fitness level increases, progressively add more difficult workouts.

3. Select a Range of Workouts: It's critical to partake in a range of workouts that focus on various muscle groups and fitness facets in order to attain complete physical wellbeing. Include cardiovascular workouts to enhance heart health and endurance, such as dance, aerobics, or running. To increase muscular strength and bone density, incorporate strength-training activities using weights or resistance bands. Remember to include stretches and yoga poses as flexibility exercises to increase joint mobility and avoid injuries.

4. Listen to Your Body: When exercising, pay attention to the cues your body gives you. It's critical to halt and rest if you feel discomfort, lightheadedness, or dyspnea. Trying to push through discomfort or agony might get you hurt. After working out, it's common to have some muscular soreness.

However, if the discomfort is severe or lasts more than a few days, you should consult a doctor.

5. Warm-up and cool-down: Make sure you always begin and conclude your workouts with an appropriate warm-up and cool-down. By boosting body temperature and enhancing blood flow to the muscles, a warm-up gets your body ready for exercise. It may consist of dynamic stretches and mild aerobic workouts. Muscle stiffness may be avoided, and your body can more easily return to a resting condition after activity by cooling down. It may entail deep breathing techniques and mild stretching.

6. Refuel Your Body and Stay Hydrated: To sustain peak performance and avoid dehydration, adequate hydration is crucial throughout exercise. Before, during, and after your workouts, sip water. To complement your training regimen, provide your body with a balanced meal rich in different nutrients. For individualized nutritional advice, speak with a dietitian or nutritionist.

7. Pay Attention to Your Body's Needs for Rest and Recovery: An essential part of any fitness regimen is rest and recovery. In order to avoid overtraining and lower your chance of injury, give your body time to rest and recuperate in between sessions. To aid your body's healing process, try to have one or two days off each week and make sure you get enough good sleep.

Part V: Survivorship and Beyond

Life After Cancer

Coping with Survivorship Challenges

Survivorship is a term used to describe life after cancer treatment. While completing treatment is a significant milestone, it is important to acknowledge that the journey doesn't end there. Many cancer survivors face unique challenges and adjustments as they navigate through the post-treatment phase. In this article, we will explore some of the common challenges faced by cancer survivors and provide coping strategies to help them thrive in their lives beyond cancer.

1. Emotional and Psychological Challenges:

After the intense physical and emotional rollercoaster of cancer treatment, many survivors experience a range of emotions, including fear, anxiety, uncertainty, and sadness. It is normal to have mixed feelings about the future and worry about the possibility of cancer recurrence. Coping with these emotions can be challenging, but there are strategies to help navigate through them. Seeking support from friends, family, or support groups, engaging in stress-reducing activities like meditation or counseling, and practicing self-care can all contribute to emotional healing and well-being.

2. Physical Changes and Side Effects:

Cancer treatment can often result in physical changes and lingering side effects that can impact a survivor's quality of life. These may include fatigue, pain, neuropathy, lymphedema, weight changes, or sexual health issues. It is important for survivors to communicate openly with their healthcare team about these concerns. They can provide guidance, recommend appropriate interventions or therapies, and help manage the side effects effectively. Engaging in regular exercise, adopting a balanced diet, and maintaining a healthy lifestyle can also contribute to overall physical well-being.

3. Rebuilding Relationships and Social Support:

During cancer treatment, relationships may have undergone strain or change due to the demands of the illness. After treatment, it is essential to rebuild and nurture relationships with loved ones, friends, and support networks. Open communication, expressing needs and concerns, and seeking professional help if necessary can facilitate the process of rebuilding relationships. Joining support groups or connecting with other cancer survivors can also provide a sense of community and understanding.

4. Fear of Recurrence and Survivor's Guilt:

The fear of cancer recurrence is a common concern among survivors. It is important to acknowledge these feelings and find healthy ways to cope with them. Engaging in activities that bring joy and a sense of purpose, focusing on self-care, and maintaining regular follow-up appointments with healthcare providers can provide reassurance. Survivor's guilt—feeling guilty for surviving when others did not—is also a common emotional challenge. Sharing feelings with trusted individuals or seeking professional support can help navigate through these complex emotions.

5. Finding Meaning and Purpose:

Surviving cancer often leads individuals to reevaluate their life's purpose and find new meaning. It can be an opportunity for

personal growth and self-discovery.
Engaging in activities that bring joy and
fulfillment, setting new goals, and exploring
new interests or hobbies can help survivors
find a renewed sense of purpose and
direction in their lives.

6. Redefining Identity:

Cancer can significantly impact a person's
identity. After treatment, survivors may
struggle with redefining themselves beyond
their cancer diagnosis. It is important to
acknowledge and embrace the new identity,
focusing on strengths and resilience.
Engaging in self-reflection, practicing
self-compassion, and seeking professional
help if needed can aid in the process of
redefining one's identity.

Emotional and Psychological Support

After cancer therapy comes a transforming phase called "survivorship." Even after active treatment comes to an end, it's critical to acknowledge that a cancer survivor's emotional and psychological health are still very essential parts of their journey. In this post, we'll discuss the value of emotional and psychological support for cancer patients and offer some coping mechanisms for when difficulties come up both during and after treatment.

1. Acknowledging and Validating Emotions: Being a cancer survivor can cause a variety of feelings, such as relief, fear, worry, thankfulness, and loss. It is critical that survivors recognize and give meaning to these feelings. It may be cathartic and help with emotional healing to give oneself permission to feel and express themselves in a secure and encouraging setting. Keeping a journal, speaking with dependable family members or friends, or obtaining professional therapy can all be beneficial for processing and controlling these feelings.

2. Making Connections with Support Networks: Having a robust support system is essential to emotional health throughout survival. Establishing relationships with fellow cancer survivors or becoming a member of support groups helps foster a feeling of belonging and empathy. Social networking sites and online discussion boards can provide opportunities to interact with people who have gone through similar things. It may be reassuring and empowering to share experiences, lessons learned, and coping mechanisms.

3. Seeking Professional Assistance: Cancer may have a profound and debilitating emotional and psychological toll. Expert advice and help can be obtained from therapists, psychologists, or counselors with a focus on cancer survival. They can assist survivors in overcoming obstacles, creating coping mechanisms, and taking care of any underlying mental health issues. Therapy sessions can provide a secure environment for processing feelings, examining personal development, and building resilience.

4. Putting Self-Care First: Making self-care a priority is crucial for emotional health throughout survival. Taking part in enjoyable, stress-relieving, and fulfilling activities can help reduce tension and foster emotional resilience. This might involve indulging in hobbies, going on nature walks, practicing mindfulness or meditation, working out frequently, getting enough rest, and eating a balanced diet. Taking care of oneself is not selfish; rather, it is an essential component of promoting emotional health.

5. Adopting Mind-Body Methods:

Mind-body methods, including yoga, deep breathing exercises, and meditation, can help with stress and anxiety management as well as improve mental health in general. These techniques foster inner peace, relaxation, and enhanced self-awareness. Many options are accessible, such as apps, online courses, and community organizations in your area that provide yoga or guided meditation programs designed especially for cancer survivors.

6. Fostering optimistic thoughts:

Emotional health may be greatly impacted by cultivating an optimistic outlook. Although negative or anxious periods are normal, practicing positive affirmations, actively cultivating appreciation, and having positive self-talk may help change viewpoints and build resilience. Keeping a good view of life may also be achieved by surrounding oneself with inspiring people and partaking in joyful and inspiring activities.

Conclusion

Looking Towards the Future

Advances in Cancer Research

Millions of individuals worldwide are impacted by the complicated and multidimensional disease known as cancer. Research on cancer has advanced significantly over time, improving survival rates, diagnosis, and therapy. In this piece, we'll look at some of the most exciting developments in cancer research recently and upcoming therapies that show promise. We will also talk about the prospects for cancer research and how they could affect cancer survivorship, treatment, and prevention in the future.

1. Immunotherapy, a form of treatment that works by stimulating the immune system to combat cancer cells. New medications that target certain proteins on cancer cells have been developed as a result of recent advancements in immunotherapy. These treatments enable the immune system to identify and combat cancer cells. The use of immunotherapy in the treatment of melanoma, lung cancer, and bladder cancer has demonstrated encouraging outcomes.

2. Precision Medicine: This method of treating cancer involves using genetic testing to find certain mutations in cancer cells. This enables medical professionals to customize treatment regimens based on each patient's unique genetic composition, improving therapeutic efficacy and minimizing adverse effects. Treatment outcomes for leukemia, lung cancer, and breast cancer with precision medicine are encouraging.

3. Liquid Biopsies: By examining blood samples for cancer cells or DNA fragments, liquid biopsies are a non-invasive technique for identifying cancer. With the use of this technology, cancer diagnosis and tracking might be completely transformed, enabling earlier identification and more individualized treatment regimens.

4. Gene editing: Using this technology, researchers may alter the genes of live cells. New gene editing techniques have made it possible to create treatments that directly target cancer cells while sparing healthy ones. Treatment of leukemia and other blood malignancies with this strategy has demonstrated encouraging outcomes.

Promising Treatments on the Horizon

1. T-cell CAR therapy:
Immunotherapy, known as CAR T-cell treatment, entails genetically altering a patient's T-cells to enable them to identify and combat cancer cells. This treatment is now being investigated for use in treating various forms of cancer, since it has had encouraging results in treating lymphoma and leukemia.

2. Nanoparticle Therapy: This technique lowers side effects and boosts treatment efficacy by employing microscopic particles to deliver medications straight to cancer cells. Treatment outcomes for pancreatic, lung, and breast cancers have been encouraging with this strategy.

3. Cancer vaccinations: A kind of immunotherapy, cancer vaccinations prime the body to identify and combat cancerous cells. New treatments that target certain proteins on cancer cells have been developed as a result of recent advancements in cancer vaccines, which improve therapeutic efficacy and minimize adverse effects.

3. Artificial Intelligence: Research and therapy for cancer might be transformed by artificial intelligence (AI). Large data sets may be analyzed by AI algorithms, which can also spot trends that human researchers would overlook. The creation of novel treatments and more individualized treatment regimens might result from this technology.